7 DAYS FULL-BODY DETOX DIET

Revitalize your body in just 7-days. Transformative detox diet for total wellness. Discover the ultimate plan for cleansing, rejuvenation and renew vitality

Odesa Mulan

Table of Content

COPYRIGHT © 2023

CHAPTER ONE

Introduction to the 7-Day Full Body Detox Diet

Embarking on a 7-day full body detox diet is a transformative journey towards revitalizing your body, mind, and spirit. In today's fast-paced world, where processed foods, environmental toxins, and stress abound, our bodies often struggle to maintain optimal health. A detox diet offers a structured approach to cleanse the body of accumulated toxins, reset dietary habits, and kick start a healthier lifestyle.

Understanding the Concept of Detoxification

Before delving into the specifics of the 7-day full body detox diet, it's crucial to grasp the concept of detoxification. Detoxification is the natural process by which the body eliminates toxins and waste products, primarily through the liver, kidneys, skin, lungs, and lymphatic system. However, due to the overwhelming burden of toxins from pollutants, pesticides, additives in food, and other sources, our bodies may become overwhelmed, leading to various health issues.

Goals and Benefits of a 7-Day Full Body Detox Diet

The primary goal of a 7-day full body detox diet is to support the body's natural detoxification processes while providing essential nutrients for optimal functioning. By eliminating processed foods, sugar, caffeine, alcohol, and other potential toxins, and focusing on whole, nutrient-dense foods, this dietary approach aims to:

1. **Eliminate Toxins:** By avoiding processed foods and minimizing exposure to environmental toxins, the body can effectively eliminate accumulated toxins, promoting overall health and vitality.

2. **Reset Eating Habits:** A detox diet serves as a reset button for unhealthy eating habits, helping individuals break free from cravings for sugar, caffeine, and junk food while fostering a preference for nourishing, whole foods.

3. **Boost Energy Levels:** By providing the body with nutrient-rich foods and reducing the burden of toxins, a detox diet can enhance energy levels, mental clarity, and overall vitality.

4. **Support Weight Loss:** Many individuals experience weight loss as a natural outcome of a detox diet, as it typically involves consuming fewer calories while focusing on nutrient-dense foods, promoting fat loss and lean muscle retention.

5. **Improve Digestive Health:** By eliminating processed foods and potential allergens, a detox diet can alleviate digestive issues such as bloating, gas, constipation, and indigestion, promoting gut health and regularity.

6. **Enhance Immune Function:** A well-nourished body with reduced toxin exposure is better equipped to support a robust immune system, reducing the risk of illness and promoting overall resilience.

7. **Promote Mental Clarity and Emotional Well-being:** Alongside physical benefits, a detox diet can also have profound effects on mental clarity and emotional well-being, reducing brain fog, improving mood stability, and fostering a sense of calm and balance.

Key Principles of the 7-Day Full Body Detox Diet

While the specifics of a detox diet may vary depending on individual needs and preferences, there are several key principles that typically characterize a 7-day full body detox:

1. **Hydration:** Adequate hydration is essential for supporting the body's detoxification processes. Drinking plenty of water throughout the day helps flush out toxins, hydrate cells, and maintain optimal bodily functions.

2. **Whole, Plant-Based Foods:** A detox diet prioritizes whole, nutrient-dense foods, with an emphasis on fruits, vegetables, leafy greens, nuts, seeds, legumes, and whole grains. These foods are rich in vitamins, minerals, antioxidants, and fiber, supporting detoxification and overall health.

3. **Elimination of Toxins:** During the detox period, it's essential to eliminate processed foods, refined sugars, artificial additives, caffeine, alcohol, and other potential toxins that burden the body and hinder its ability to detoxify effectively.

4. **Supportive Nutrients:** Incorporating foods rich in detox-supportive nutrients such as antioxidants (e.g., vitamin C, vitamin E, selenium), sulfur (found in garlic, onions, cruciferous vegetables), and fiber (found in fruits, vegetables, whole grains) can enhance the body's detoxification pathways.

5. **Gentle Exercise:** Engaging in gentle exercise such as walking, yoga, or stretching can support lymphatic drainage, circulation, and overall well-being during the detox process.

6. **Stress Management:** Stress can impede the body's detoxification efforts, so incorporating stress-reducing practices such as meditation, deep breathing exercises, or mindfulness can complement the detox diet and promote relaxation.

7. **Adequate Rest and Sleep:** Prioritizing sufficient rest and quality sleep is essential for allowing the body to repair, regenerate, and detoxify efficiently.

Sample Meal Plan for a 7-Day Full Body Detox Diet

A sample meal plan for a 7-day full body detox diet might include:

Day 1:

- Breakfast: Green smoothie (spinach, kale, banana, avocado, almond milk)

- Snack: Apple slices with almond butter

- Lunch: Quinoa salad with mixed vegetables (bell peppers, cucumber, cherry tomatoes, avocado) and lemon-tahini dressing

- Snack: Carrot sticks with hummus

- Dinner: Baked salmon with steamed broccoli and quinoa

Day 2:

- Breakfast: Chia seed pudding topped with mixed berries and chopped nuts

- Snack: Celery sticks with guacamole

- Lunch: Lentil soup with a side of mixed greens salad (lettuce, cucumber, radishes, balsamic vinaigrette)

- Snack: Raw almonds and dried apricots

- Dinner: Stir-fried tofu with vegetables (bell peppers, broccoli, snow peas) served over brown rice

Day 3:

- Breakfast: Overnight oats with almond milk, sliced banana, and cinnamon
- Snack: Greek yogurt with honey and sliced strawberries
- Lunch: Chickpea salad with mixed greens, cherry tomatoes, cucumbers, and lemon-tahini dressing
- Snack: Rice cakes with mashed avocado and cherry tomatoes
- Dinner: Grilled chicken breast with roasted sweet potatoes and steamed asparagus

Day 4:

- Breakfast: Acai bowl topped with granola, sliced kiwi, and coconut flakes
- Snack: Mixed nuts and dried cranberries
- Lunch: Quinoa and black bean stuffed bell peppers with a side of mixed greens salad
- Snack: Sliced cucumber with hummus
- Dinner: Baked cod with roasted Brussels sprouts and quinoa pilaf

Day 5:

- Breakfast: Spinach and mushroom omelet with whole grain toast

- Snack: Orange slices

- Lunch: Vegetable stir-fry with tofu or tempeh served over brown rice

- Snack: Rice cakes with almond butter and banana slices

- Dinner: Zucchini noodles with marinara sauce and grilled shrimp

Day 6:

- Breakfast: Berry smoothie bowl topped with sliced almonds and shredded coconut

- Snack: Edamame pods

- Lunch: Lentil and vegetable curry with a side of steamed basmati rice

- Snack: Bell pepper strips with hummus

- Dinner: Baked turkey meatballs with spaghetti squash and marinara sauce

Day 7:

- Breakfast: Avocado toast on whole grain bread with cherry tomatoes and microgreens

- Snack: Trail mix with assorted nuts and seeds

- Lunch: Quinoa and roasted vegetable salad with lemon-tahini dressing

- Snack: Sliced cucumber with tzatziki sauce

- Dinner: Grilled salmon with steamed green beans and wild rice pilaf

Conclusion

Embarking on a 7-day full body detox diet can be a powerful way to jumpstart your journey towards improved health and well-being. By prioritizing whole, nutrient-dense foods, eliminating toxins, and supporting the body's natural detoxification processes, you can experience a myriad of benefits, including increased energy, improved digestion, enhanced immune function, and mental clarity. Remember to listen to your body, stay hydrated, and incorporate stress-reducing practices for a holistic approach to detoxification and overall wellness.

CHAPTER TWO

Understanding the Benefits of a Full Body Detox

Embarking on a full body detox can be a profound journey towards rejuvenating your physical, mental, and emotional well-being. In a world filled with environmental toxins, processed foods, and daily stressors, our bodies can become overwhelmed, leading to a range of health issues. By engaging in a comprehensive detoxification process, individuals can experience a wide array of benefits that extend beyond mere physical cleansing.

1. Elimination of Toxins

One of the primary benefits of a full body detox is the elimination of accumulated toxins from the body. Toxins can enter our system through various sources, including pollution, pesticides in food, household chemicals, and even stress. Over time, these toxins can build up in our organs and tissues, impairing their function and contributing to chronic health conditions. A thorough detoxification process helps flush out these toxins, allowing the body to function optimally and reducing the risk of illness.

2. Improved Digestive Health

Many detox programs emphasize the consumption of whole, nutrient-dense foods and the elimination of processed foods and allergens. This dietary shift can have a significant impact on digestive health. By removing foods that may cause inflammation or irritation in the gut, such as gluten, dairy, and refined sugars, and replacing them with fiber-rich fruits, vegetables, and whole grains, individuals may experience relief from digestive issues such as bloating, gas, constipation, and indigestion. Additionally, detox diets often include probiotic-rich foods that support the growth of beneficial gut bacteria, further enhancing digestive function.

3. Increased Energy and Vitality

As the body eliminates toxins and receives nourishment from nutrient-dense foods during a detox, many individuals report experiencing increased energy levels and vitality. Without the burden of processed foods and toxins, the body can more efficiently convert nutrients into energy, leading to a greater sense of vitality and well-being. This surge in energy can translate into improved productivity, enhanced physical performance, and a greater capacity to engage in activities that bring joy and fulfillment.

4. Weight Loss and Body Composition Improvement

For some individuals, a full body detox can lead to weight loss and improvements in body composition. By eliminating processed foods, refined sugars, and excess calories, and focusing on whole, nutrient-dense foods, individuals may naturally reduce their calorie intake and shed excess fat. Additionally, detox diets often emphasize hydration, which can help reduce water retention and bloating. As individuals adopt healthier eating habits and engage in regular physical activity during the detox process, they may experience sustainable weight loss and improvements in muscle tone and definition.

5. Enhanced Immune Function

A well-functioning immune system is essential for protecting the body against infections and illnesses. By supporting the body's natural detoxification processes and providing it with essential nutrients, a full body detox can enhance immune function. Nutrient-dense foods such as fruits, vegetables, nuts, seeds, and lean proteins provide the vitamins, minerals, antioxidants, and phytonutrients necessary for optimal immune function. Additionally, reducing the burden of toxins on the body allows the immune system to focus its resources on combating pathogens and maintaining health.

6. Mental Clarity and Emotional Well-being

In addition to physical benefits, a full body detox can also have profound effects on mental clarity and emotional well-being. Many individuals report feeling more focused, alert, and mentally sharp during and after a detox. This may be attributed to factors such as improved digestion, balanced blood sugar levels, and reduced inflammation, all of which can positively impact brain function. Furthermore, the dietary changes and lifestyle practices associated with a detox, such as mindfulness, stress reduction, and adequate sleep, can promote emotional balance, reduce anxiety and depression, and foster a greater sense of inner peace and well-being.

7. Establishment of Healthy Habits

Perhaps one of the most significant benefits of a full body detox is the establishment of healthy habits that can be sustained long after the detox period ends. By experiencing firsthand the positive effects of nourishing foods, regular exercise, adequate hydration, and stress management techniques, individuals are often motivated to continue prioritizing their health and well-being beyond the duration of the detox. This can lead to lasting lifestyle changes, such as adopting a predominantly plant-based diet, engaging in regular physical activity, practicing mindfulness, and avoiding toxins in everyday products.

In conclusion, the benefits of a full body detox extend far beyond physical cleansing. By supporting the body's natural detoxification processes, improving digestive health, boosting energy levels, promoting weight loss, enhancing immune function, fostering mental clarity and emotional well-being, and establishing healthy habits, individuals can experience a comprehensive transformation that encompasses mind, body, and spirit. Whether undertaken as a short-term cleanse or as part of a long-term wellness strategy, a full body detox has the potential to profoundly improve overall health and vitality.

CHAPTER THREE

Preparing Mentally and Physically for the Detox

Embarking on a detox journey requires thorough preparation both mentally and physically to ensure a successful and sustainable experience. By taking the time to prepare adequately, individuals can optimize their detoxification process, minimize potential challenges, and set themselves up for long-term success. Here's a detailed guide on how to prepare mentally and physically for a detox:

1. Set Clear Intentions

Before beginning the detox, take some time to reflect on your reasons for doing it and set clear intentions for what you hope to achieve. Whether your goals include improving energy levels, supporting digestive health, or breaking unhealthy eating habits, clarifying your intentions will provide you with a sense of purpose and motivation throughout the process.

2. Educate Yourself

Educate yourself about the detox process, including what to expect, common challenges, and potential benefits. Understanding the rationale behind the detox and how it can positively impact your health will help you stay committed and motivated, especially when faced with obstacles along the way.

3. Consult with a Healthcare Professional

Before starting any detox program, it's essential to consult with a healthcare professional, especially if you have any underlying health conditions or are taking medications. A healthcare provider can offer personalized guidance, ensure the detox is safe for you, and address any concerns or questions you may have.

4. Gradually Reduce Toxins

In the days leading up to the detox, gradually reduce your intake of toxins such as caffeine, alcohol, processed foods, and refined sugars. This gradual approach can help minimize withdrawal symptoms and make the transition into the detox smoother.

5. Plan Your Meals

Take the time to plan your meals for the duration of the detox, ensuring they are balanced, nutrient-dense, and aligned with the detox guidelines. Consider incorporating a variety of fruits, vegetables, whole grains, lean proteins, and healthy fats to provide your body with essential nutrients and support its detoxification processes.

6. Stock Up on Supplies

Ensure you have all the necessary supplies and ingredients for your detox, including fresh produce, whole grains, legumes, nuts, seeds, and any supplements or detox aids you plan to use. Having everything you need on hand will make it easier to stick to your detox plan and avoid temptation.

7. Clear Your Schedule

Try to clear your schedule as much as possible during the detox period to minimize stress and allow yourself time to focus on self-care. Consider scheduling lighter workloads, reducing social commitments, and prioritizing activities that promote relaxation and well-being.

8. Practice Mindfulness and Stress Reduction

Incorporate mindfulness practices and stress reduction techniques into your daily routine to support your mental and emotional well-being during the detox. This may include meditation, deep breathing exercises, yoga, journaling, or spending time in nature. These practices can help reduce stress levels, promote relaxation, and enhance your overall detox experience.

9. Stay Hydrated

Hydration is essential for supporting the body's detoxification processes, so make sure to drink plenty of water throughout the day. Consider adding herbal teas, lemon water, or infused water to your hydration routine for added flavor and benefits.

10. Get Adequate Rest and Sleep

Prioritize getting adequate rest and sleep during the detox period to allow your body time to repair, regenerate, and detoxify. Aim for seven to nine hours of quality sleep per night and incorporate relaxation techniques before bedtime to promote restful sleep.

11. Seek Support

Lastly, seek support from friends, family, or online communities who can offer encouragement, accountability, and guidance throughout your detox journey. Having a support system in place can make a significant difference in your ability to stay motivated and committed to your goals.

By following these steps to prepare mentally and physically for a detox, you can set yourself up for a successful and transformative experience. Remember to approach the process with patience, self-compassion, and an open mind, allowing yourself to embrace the journey and all its potential benefits.

CHAPTER FOUR

The Science Behind Detoxification: How It Works

Detoxification is a complex physiological process through which the body eliminates toxins and waste products to maintain homeostasis and promote optimal health. It involves various organs, systems, and biochemical pathways working together to identify, neutralize, and excrete harmful substances from the body. Understanding the science behind detoxification can provide insights into how this vital process works and how it can be supported through lifestyle choices and dietary interventions.

1. Liver Detoxification

The liver plays a central role in detoxification, serving as the primary organ responsible for processing and neutralizing toxins. The liver performs two main phases of detoxification: Phase I and Phase II.

Phase I Detoxification: During Phase I, enzymes known as cytochrome P450 enzymes catalyze chemical reactions that transform fat-soluble toxins into intermediate metabolites. These metabolites are often more reactive and potentially harmful than the original toxins, making Phase II detoxification essential for their safe elimination.

Phase II Detoxification: In Phase II, conjugation reactions occur, in which the intermediate metabolites produced in Phase I are combined with water-soluble molecules to render them less toxic and more easily excreted from the body. Conjugation reactions involve various pathways, including glutathione conjugation, amino acid conjugation, methylation, sulfation, and glucuronidation.

Once toxins have undergone Phase II detoxification, they are typically converted into water-soluble compounds that can be eliminated from the body via urine, bile, sweat, or feces.

2. Kidney Filtration

The kidneys play a crucial role in detoxification by filtering waste products and toxins from the blood and excreting them in the form of urine. The kidneys contain millions of nephrons, which are microscopic units responsible for filtering blood and regulating the body's fluid balance, electrolyte levels, and pH.

Toxins that have been processed by the liver and rendered water-soluble are filtered out of the bloodstream by the kidneys and excreted in urine. Adequate hydration is essential for supporting kidney function and ensuring the efficient elimination of toxins.

3. Lymphatic System

The lymphatic system is another key component of the body's detoxification pathways. It consists of a network of vessels and lymph nodes that help remove toxins, waste products, and pathogens from the body's tissues and transport them to lymph nodes, where they are filtered and destroyed.

Unlike the circulatory system, which is powered by the heart, the lymphatic system relies on muscle contractions, breathing, and physical movement to circulate lymph fluid throughout the body. Engaging in regular exercise, massage, dry brushing, and lymphatic drainage techniques can help stimulate lymphatic flow and support detoxification.

4. Skin Detoxification

The skin, the body's largest organ, also plays a role in detoxification through the process of sweating. Sweat glands in the skin help eliminate toxins and waste products from the body by excreting them through sweat. Sweating is a natural response to physical exertion, heat, stress, and other factors that increase body temperature.

Saunas, steam baths, hot yoga, and vigorous exercise are all activities that promote sweating and support skin detoxification. Additionally, dry brushing and exfoliation can help remove dead skin cells and unclog pores, allowing toxins to be released more effectively through the skin.

5. Gut Detoxification

The gastrointestinal tract, or gut, is involved in detoxification through the process of digestion and elimination. The gut serves as a barrier between the internal environment of the body and the external environment, helping to prevent the absorption of harmful substances into the bloodstream.

Fiber-rich foods such as fruits, vegetables, whole grains, and legumes support gut health and regular bowel movements, facilitating the elimination of toxins from the body. Additionally, the gut microbiota, consisting of trillions of beneficial bacteria, plays a crucial role in detoxification by metabolizing dietary fibers, producing essential nutrients, and modulating immune function.

6. Antioxidant Defense

Antioxidants are molecules that help neutralize free radicals and protect cells from oxidative damage caused by toxins, pollutants, and metabolic byproducts. Many antioxidants are found naturally in fruits, vegetables, nuts, seeds, and spices, and they play a vital role in supporting the body's detoxification pathways.

Key antioxidants involved in detoxification include vitamin C, vitamin E, glutathione, selenium, and phytonutrients such as flavonoids, carotenoids, and polyphenols. These antioxidants help quench free radicals, regenerate other antioxidants, and enhance the body's ability to neutralize and eliminate toxins.

In conclusion, detoxification is a multifaceted process that involves the liver, kidneys, lymphatic system, skin, gut, and antioxidant defenses working together to eliminate toxins and waste products from the body. By understanding the science behind detoxification and supporting the body's natural detoxification pathways through lifestyle choices, dietary interventions, and targeted therapies, individuals can optimize their health and well-being and reduce the burden of environmental toxins on the body.

CHAPTER FIVE

Essential Foods for Detoxification and Cleansing

When embarking on a detoxification and cleansing journey, choosing the right foods is essential for supporting the body's natural detoxification processes and promoting overall health and vitality. Incorporating nutrient-dense, whole foods rich in antioxidants, vitamins, minerals, fiber, and phytonutrients can help nourish the body, eliminate toxins, and optimize detoxification pathways. Here's a comprehensive list of essential foods for detoxification and cleansing:

1. Leafy Greens

Leafy greens such as spinach, kale, Swiss chard, collard greens, and arugula are powerhouse foods for detoxification. Rich in chlorophyll, vitamins (such as vitamin A, vitamin C, and vitamin K), minerals (including magnesium, potassium, and calcium), and antioxidants, leafy greens support liver function, promote alkalinity, and aid in the elimination of toxins from the body.

2. Cruciferous Vegetables

Cruciferous vegetables such as broccoli, cauliflower, Brussels sprouts, cabbage, and kale contain compounds known as glucosinolates, which support detoxification pathways in the liver. These vegetables are also rich in fiber, vitamins, minerals, and antioxidants, making them excellent choices for cleansing and supporting overall health.

3. Berries

Berries such as blueberries, strawberries, raspberries, and blackberries are loaded with antioxidants, including anthocyanins, flavonoids, and vitamin C. These antioxidants help neutralize free radicals, reduce inflammation, and support cellular health. Berries are also low in sugar and high in fiber, making them an ideal choice for cleansing and detoxification.

4. Citrus Fruits

Citrus fruits such as lemons, limes, oranges, and grapefruits are rich in vitamin C and other antioxidants that support liver detoxification and boost immune function. Drinking warm lemon water in the morning is a popular practice for stimulating digestion, hydrating the body, and promoting detoxification.

5. Cruciferous Sprouts

Cruciferous sprouts such as broccoli sprouts, radish sprouts, and alfalfa sprouts are concentrated sources of nutrients and phytonutrients that support detoxification. Sprouts contain high levels of glucosinolates and sulforaphane, compounds known for their potent antioxidant and detoxifying properties.

6. Garlic and Onions

Garlic and onions are members of the allium family and are rich in sulfur-containing compounds that support liver detoxification and enhance the body's ability to eliminate toxins. These pungent vegetables also have antimicrobial and anti-inflammatory properties, making them valuable additions to a detox diet.

7. Turmeric

Turmeric, a bright yellow spice commonly used in Indian cuisine, contains a compound called curcumin, which has powerful anti-inflammatory and antioxidant properties. Curcumin supports liver function, promotes bile production, and helps neutralize toxins in the body.

8. Ginger

Ginger is well-known for its digestive benefits and is often used to alleviate nausea, bloating, and indigestion. It also has anti-inflammatory and antioxidant properties that support detoxification and promote overall health. Drinking ginger tea or adding fresh ginger to smoothies and dishes can help support cleansing and detoxification.

9. Green Tea

Green tea is rich in antioxidants called catechins, which have been shown to support liver function and promote detoxification. Drinking green tea regularly can help boost metabolism, improve fat metabolism, and support weight loss efforts during a detox.

10. Nuts and Seeds

Nuts and seeds such as almonds, walnuts, chia seeds, and flaxseeds are excellent sources of healthy fats, fiber, protein, vitamins, and minerals. These nutrient-dense foods support satiety, regulate blood sugar levels, and provide essential nutrients needed for detoxification and overall health.

11. Legumes

Legumes such as lentils, chickpeas, black beans, and kidney beans are rich in fiber, protein, vitamins, and minerals. They help stabilize blood sugar levels, support digestive health, and provide sustained energy for detoxification and cleansing.

12. Whole Grains

Whole grains such as quinoa, brown rice, oats, and barley are rich in fiber, vitamins, minerals, and antioxidants. They provide sustained energy, promote satiety, and support digestive health, making them valuable additions to a detox diet.

13. Fermented Foods

Fermented foods such as yogurt, kefir, sauerkraut, kimchi, and kombucha contain beneficial probiotics that support gut health and digestion. A healthy gut microbiome is essential for detoxification and overall well-being, as it helps eliminate toxins, produce essential nutrients, and regulate immune function.

14. Herbs and Spices

Herbs and spices such as cilantro, parsley, dandelion greens, mint, and cinnamon have detoxifying properties and can be easily incorporated into meals, smoothies, and teas. These flavorful additions not only enhance the taste of dishes but also provide additional nutrients and support detoxification pathways in the body.

15. Water

Last but not least, staying hydrated is crucial for supporting detoxification and cleansing. Drinking an adequate amount of water helps flush out toxins, maintain electrolyte balance, support kidney function, and promote overall health. Aim to drink at least eight glasses of water per day, or more if you're engaging in vigorous physical activity or sweating heavily.

Incorporating these essential foods into your diet can help support detoxification and cleansing, promote overall health and vitality, and enhance your well-being from the inside out. Remember to focus on whole, nutrient-dense foods, minimize processed foods and refined sugars, and listen to your body's signals to ensure a safe and effective detoxification experience.

CHAPTER SIX

7-Day Detox Meal Plan and Recipes

Embarking on a 7-day detox journey requires careful planning and preparation to ensure you nourish your body with nutrient-dense foods while supporting its natural detoxification processes. Below is a sample meal plan for each day of the detox, along with delicious recipes to help you stay on track and feel your best throughout the week.

Day 1: Cleanse and Energize

Breakfast: Green Smoothie

Ingredients:

- 1 cup spinach

- 1/2 cucumber

- 1/2 green apple

- 1/2 banana

- 1 tablespoon fresh lemon juice

- 1 cup coconut water

- Ice cubes (optional)

Instructions:

1. Add all ingredients to a blender.

2. Blend until smooth and creamy.

3. Pour into a glass and enjoy!

Lunch: Quinoa Salad with Chickpeas and Veggies

Ingredients:

- 1 cup cooked quinoa

- 1/2 cup cooked chickpeas

- 1/2 cup cherry tomatoes, halved

- 1/2 cucumber, diced

- 1/4 red onion, thinly sliced

- 1/4 cup chopped fresh parsley

- Juice of 1 lemon

- 2 tablespoons extra virgin olive oil

- Salt and pepper to taste

Instructions:

1. In a large bowl, combine quinoa, chickpeas, cherry tomatoes, cucumber, red onion, and parsley.

2. Drizzle with lemon juice and olive oil.

3. Season with salt and pepper to taste.

4. Toss until well combined.

5. Serve chilled or at room temperature.

Dinner: Baked Salmon with Steamed Broccoli

Ingredients:

- 2 salmon fillets
- 1 tablespoon olive oil
- 1 teaspoon lemon zest
- 1 teaspoon minced garlic
- 1/2 teaspoon dried dill
- Salt and pepper to taste
- 2 cups broccoli florets

Instructions:

1. Preheat the oven to 375°F (190°C).
2. Place salmon fillets on a baking sheet lined with parchment paper.
3. In a small bowl, whisk together olive oil, lemon zest, minced garlic, dried dill, salt, and pepper.
4. Brush the salmon fillets with the olive oil mixture.
5. Bake for 12-15 minutes, or until salmon is cooked through and flakes easily with a fork.

6. While the salmon is baking, steam broccoli florets until tender.

7. Serve the baked salmon with steamed broccoli on the side.

Day 2: Revitalize with Fresh Flavors

Breakfast: Berry Chia Seed Pudding

Ingredients:

- 1/4 cup chia seeds

- 1 cup unsweetened almond milk

- 1/2 teaspoon pure vanilla extract

- 1 tablespoon maple syrup (optional)

- 1/2 cup mixed berries (such as strawberries, blueberries, raspberries)

Instructions:

1. In a jar or bowl, combine chia seeds, almond milk, vanilla extract, and maple syrup (if using).

2. Stir well to combine.

3. Cover and refrigerate for at least 2 hours or overnight, until the chia seeds have absorbed the liquid and formed a pudding-like consistency.

4. Before serving, top with mixed berries.

Lunch: Lentil and Vegetable Soup

Ingredients:

- 1 tablespoon olive oil
- 1 onion, diced
- 2 carrots, diced
- 2 celery stalks, diced
- 2 cloves garlic, minced
- 1 cup dried green lentils, rinsed and drained
- 4 cups vegetable broth
- 1 teaspoon dried thyme
- 1 bay leaf
- Salt and pepper to taste
- Fresh parsley for garnish (optional)

Instructions:

1. In a large pot, heat olive oil over medium heat.
2. Add diced onion, carrots, celery, and garlic. Cook until vegetables are softened, about 5 minutes.
3. Add dried lentils, vegetable broth, dried thyme, and bay leaf.

4. Bring to a boil, then reduce heat and simmer for 20-25 minutes, or until lentils are tender.

5. Season with salt and pepper to taste.

6. Serve hot, garnished with fresh parsley if desired.

Dinner: Vegetable Stir-Fry with Tofu

Ingredients:

- 8 ounces extra-firm tofu, pressed and cubed

- 2 tablespoons soy sauce or tamari

- 1 tablespoon sesame oil

- 1 tablespoon olive oil

- 2 cups mixed vegetables (such as bell peppers, broccoli, carrots, snap peas)

- 2 cloves garlic, minced

- 1 tablespoon grated ginger

- Cooked brown rice for serving

Instructions:

1. In a small bowl, marinate cubed tofu in soy sauce or tamari for 15-20 minutes.

2. In a large skillet or wok, heat olive oil and sesame oil over medium-high heat.

3. Add marinated tofu and cook until golden brown on all sides, about 5 minutes. Remove from skillet and set aside.

4. In the same skillet, add mixed vegetables, garlic, and ginger. Stir-fry until vegetables are tender-crisp, about 5-7 minutes.

5. Return cooked tofu to the skillet and toss to combine with the vegetables.

6. Serve vegetable stir-fry with cooked brown rice.

Day 3: Recharge with Nutrient-Rich Foods

Breakfast: Overnight Oats with Mixed Berries

Ingredients:

- 1/2 cup rolled oats

- 1/2 cup unsweetened almond milk

- 1 tablespoon chia seeds

- 1/2 teaspoon pure vanilla extract

- 1 tablespoon maple syrup (optional)

- 1/2 cup mixed berries (such as strawberries, blueberries, raspberries)

Instructions:

1. In a jar or bowl, combine rolled oats, almond milk, chia seeds, vanilla extract, and maple syrup (if using).

2. Stir well to combine.

3. Cover and refrigerate overnight.

4. Before serving, top with mixed berries.

Lunch: Chickpea and Avocado Salad

Ingredients:

- 1 can (15 ounces) chickpeas, rinsed and drained

- 1 avocado, diced

- 1/2 cucumber, diced

- 1/2 red bell pepper, diced

- 1/4 cup diced red onion

- 2 tablespoons chopped fresh cilantro or parsley

- Juice of 1 lime

- 1 tablespoon extra virgin olive oil

- Salt and pepper to taste

Instructions:

1. In a large bowl, combine chickpeas, diced avocado, cucumber, red bell pepper, red onion, and chopped cilantro or parsley.

2. Drizzle with lime juice and olive oil.

3. Season with salt and pepper to taste.

4. Toss until well combined.

5. Serve chilled or at room temperature.

Dinner: Lentil and Vegetable Curry

Ingredients:

- 1 tablespoon coconut oil

- 1 onion, diced

- 2 cloves garlic, minced

- 1 tablespoon grated ginger

- 2 tablespoons curry powder

- 1 can (14 ounces) diced tomatoes

- 1 can (14 ounces) coconut milk

- 1 cup dried red lentils, rinsed and drained

- 2 cups chopped vegetables (such as cauliflower, carrots, bell peppers)

- Salt and pepper to taste

- Fresh cilantro for garnish (optional)

Instructions:

1. In a large pot or Dutch oven, heat coconut oil over medium heat.

2. Add diced onion, garlic, and grated ginger. Cook until onion is softened, about 5 minutes.

3. Stir in curry powder and cook for an additional minute.

4. Add diced tomatoes (with their juices), coconut milk, dried red lentils, chopped vegetables, salt, and pepper.

5. Bring to a boil, then reduce heat and simmer, covered, for 20-25 minutes, or until lentils and vegetables are tender.

6. Serve hot, garnished with fresh cilantro if desired.

Day 4: Refresh with Vibrant Flavors

Breakfast: Green Detox Smoothie Bowl

Ingredients:

- 1 cup spinach

- 1/2 frozen banana

- 1/2 cup frozen mixed berries

- 1/4 avocado

- 1 tablespoon chia seeds

- 1/2 cup unsweetened almond milk

- Toppings: sliced banana, fresh berries, granola, coconut flakes

Instructions:

1. In a blender, combine spinach, frozen banana, frozen mixed berries, avocado, chia seeds, and almond milk.

2. Blend until smooth and creamy.

3. Pour into a bowl and top with sliced banana, fresh berries, granola, and coconut flakes.

Lunch: Roasted Vegetable Quinoa Bowl

Ingredients:

- 1 cup cooked quinoa

- 1 cup roasted vegetables (such as sweet potatoes, carrots, Brussels sprouts)

- 1/2 cup cooked chickpeas

- 2 tablespoons tahini

- 1 tablespoon lemon juice

- 1 clove garlic, minced

- Water (as needed)

- Salt and pepper to taste

- Fresh parsley for garnish (optional)

Instructions:

1. In a bowl, combine cooked quinoa, roasted vegetables, and cooked chickpeas.

2. In a small bowl, whisk together tahini, lemon juice, minced garlic, and water (as needed) to thin out the dressing.

3. Drizzle the tahini dressing over the quinoa bowl.

4. Season with salt and pepper to taste.

5. Garnish with fresh parsley if desired.

Dinner: Zucchini Noodles with Pesto

Ingredients:

- 2 medium zucchini

- 1/4 cup basil pesto

- Cherry tomatoes, halved (for garnish)

- Pine nuts (for garnish)

- Fresh basil leaves (for garnish)

Instructions:

1. Using a spiralizer, spiralize the zucchini into noodles.

2. In a large skillet, heat basil pesto over medium heat.

3. Add zucchini noodles to the skillet and toss to coat in the pesto.

4. Cook for 2-3 minutes, or until zucchini noodles are heated through but still crisp.

5. Transfer zucchini noodles to serving plates.

6. Garnish with cherry tomatoes, pine nuts, and fresh basil leaves.

Day 5: Renew with Plant-Based Goodness

Breakfast: Acai Bowl

Ingredients:

- 1 pack frozen unsweetened acai puree

- 1/2 frozen banana

- 1/2 cup frozen mixed berries

- 1/2 cup unsweetened almond milk

- Toppings: granola, sliced banana, fresh berries, shredded coconut

Instructions:

1. In a blender, combine frozen acai puree, frozen banana, frozen mixed berries, and almond milk.

2. Blend until smooth and creamy.

3. Pour into a bowl and top with granola, sliced banana, fresh berries, and shredded coconut.

Lunch: Mediterranean Quinoa Salad

Ingredients:

- 1 cup cooked quinoa

- 1/2 cup cherry tomatoes, halved

- 1/2 cucumber, diced

- 1/4 red onion, thinly sliced

- 1/4 cup Kalamata olives, pitted and sliced

- 2 tablespoons chopped fresh parsley

- 2 tablespoons extra virgin olive oil

- 1 tablespoon red wine vinegar

- Salt and pepper to taste

- Crumbled feta cheese (optional)

Instructions:

1. In a large bowl, combine cooked quinoa, cherry tomatoes, cucumber, red onion, Kalamata olives, and chopped parsley.

2. Drizzle with olive oil and red wine vinegar.

3. Season with salt and pepper to taste.

4. Toss until well combined.

5. Serve chilled or at room temperature, topped with crumbled feta cheese if desired.

Dinner: Cauliflower Rice Stir-Fry with Tofu

Ingredients:

- 8 ounces extra-firm tofu, pressed and cubed

- 2 tablespoons soy sauce or tamari

- 1 tablespoon sesame oil

- 1 tablespoon olive oil

- 2 cups cauliflower rice

- 1 cup mixed vegetables (such as bell peppers, broccoli, carrots, snap peas)

- 2 cloves garlic, minced

- 1 tablespoon grated ginger

- Cooked edamame for serving (optional)

Instructions:

1. In a small bowl, marinate cubed tofu in soy sauce or tamari for 15-20 minutes.

2. In a large skillet or wok, heat olive oil and sesame oil over medium-high heat.

3. Add marinated tofu and cook until golden brown on all sides, about 5 minutes. Remove from skillet and set aside.

4. In the same skillet, add cauliflower rice, mixed vegetables, garlic, and ginger. Stir-fry until vegetables are tender-crisp, about 5-7 minutes.

5. Return cooked tofu to the skillet and toss to combine with the cauliflower rice and vegetables.

6. Serve cauliflower rice stir-fry with cooked edamame on the side.

Day 6: Replenish with Whole Foods

Breakfast: Coconut Chia Pudding with Mango

Ingredients:

- 1/4 cup chia seeds

- 1 cup unsweetened coconut milk

- 1 tablespoon maple syrup (optional)

- 1/2 teaspoon pure vanilla extract

- 1/2 cup diced mango

- Toasted coconut flakes (for garnish)

Instructions:

1. In a jar or bowl, combine chia seeds, coconut milk, maple syrup (if using), and vanilla extract.

2. Stir well to combine.

3. Cover and refrigerate for at least 2 hours or overnight, until the chia seeds have absorbed the liquid and formed a pudding-like consistency.

4. Before serving, top with diced mango and toasted coconut flakes.

Lunch: Spinach and Avocado Salad with Lemon-Tahini Dressing

Ingredients:

- 2 cups baby spinach

- 1/2 avocado, diced

- 1/4 cup sliced cucumber

- 1/4 cup sliced radishes

- 2 tablespoons sunflower seeds

- Lemon-Tahini Dressing (see recipe below)

Lemon-Tahini Dressing:

- 2 tablespoons tahini

- Juice of 1 lemon

- 1 tablespoon extra virgin olive oil

- 1 teaspoon maple syrup

- 1 clove garlic, minced

- Water (as needed)

- Salt and pepper to taste

Instructions:

1. In a large bowl, combine baby spinach, diced avocado, sliced cucumber, sliced radishes, and sunflower seeds.

2. In a small bowl, whisk together tahini, lemon juice, olive oil, maple syrup, minced garlic, and water (as needed) to thin out the dressing.

3. Drizzle the lemon-tahini dressing over the salad.

4. Season with salt and pepper to taste.

5. Toss until well combined.

Dinner: Stuffed Bell Peppers with Quinoa and Black Beans

Ingredients:

- 4 bell peppers (any color), halved and seeded
- 1 cup cooked quinoa
- 1 cup cooked black beans
- 1 cup diced tomatoes
- 1/2 cup corn kernels
- 1/4 cup diced red onion
- 1/4 cup chopped fresh cilantro
- 1 teaspoon ground cumin
- 1/2 teaspoon chili powder
- Salt and pepper to taste
- Sliced avocado for serving (optional)

Instructions:

1. Preheat the oven to 375°F (190°C).
2. Place bell pepper halves in a baking dish, cut side up.
3. In a large bowl, combine cooked quinoa, cooked black beans, diced tomatoes, corn kernels, diced red onion, chopped cilantro, ground cumin, chili powder, salt, and pepper.

4. Spoon the quinoa and black bean mixture into the bell pepper halves.

5. Cover the baking dish with foil and bake for 30-35 minutes, or until the peppers are tender.

6. Serve stuffed bell peppers with sliced avocado on the side.

Day 7: Rejuvenate with Healing Foods

Breakfast: Mango Coconut Smoothie Bowl

Ingredients:

- 1/2 cup frozen mango chunks

- 1/2 frozen banana

- 1/4 cup unsweetened coconut milk

- 1/4 cup unsweetened Greek yogurt or dairy-free yogurt

- Toppings: sliced mango, shredded coconut, granola, chia seeds

Instructions:

1. In a blender, combine frozen mango chunks, frozen banana, coconut milk, and Greek yogurt.

2. Blend until smooth and creamy.

3. Pour into a bowl and top with sliced mango, shredded coconut, granola, and chia seeds.

Lunch: Detoxifying Green Soup

Ingredients:

- 1 tablespoon olive oil

- 1 onion, diced

- 2 cloves garlic, minced

- 4 cups vegetable broth

- 4 cups chopped leafy greens (such as spinach, kale, Swiss chard)

- 1 cup chopped broccoli florets

- 1 cup chopped zucchini

- 1 teaspoon dried thyme

- Salt and pepper to taste

- Fresh lemon juice for serving

- Fresh herbs for garnish (such as parsley or cilantro)

Instructions:

1. In a large pot, heat olive oil over medium heat.

2. Add diced onion and minced garlic. Cook until onion is softened, about 5 minutes.

3. Add vegetable broth, chopped leafy greens, chopped broccoli florets, chopped zucchini, dried thyme, salt, and pepper.

4. Bring to a boil, then reduce heat and simmer for 15-20 minutes, or until vegetables are tender.

5. Remove from heat and let cool slightly.

6. Using an immersion blender or regular blender, puree the soup until smooth and creamy.

7. Serve hot, garnished with fresh lemon juice and herbs.

Dinner: Baked Sweet Potato with Black Bean Salsa

Ingredients:

- 2 medium sweet potatoes
- 1 can (15 ounces) black beans, rinsed and drained
- 1/2 cup diced tomatoes
- 1/4 cup diced red onion
- 1/4 cup chopped fresh cilantro
- Juice of 1 lime
- Salt and pepper to taste
- Sliced avocado for serving (optional)

Instructions:

1. Preheat the oven to 400°F (200°C).

2. Wash sweet potatoes and prick them several times with a fork.

3. Place sweet potatoes on a baking sheet lined with parchment paper.

4. Bake for 45-60 minutes, or until sweet potatoes are tender and cooked through.

5. While sweet potatoes are baking, prepare the black bean salsa.

6. In a bowl, combine black beans, diced tomatoes, diced red onion, chopped cilantro, lime juice, salt, and pepper.

7. Once sweet potatoes are cooked, slice them open lengthwise and fluff the insides with a fork.

8. Top each sweet potato with black bean salsa and sliced avocado if desired.

Snacks and Beverages:

Throughout the day, enjoy snacks such as fresh fruit, raw vegetables with hummus, nuts, seeds, and herbal teas. Stay hydrated by drinking plenty of water, infused water, herbal teas, and green juices.

Important Notes:

- Listen to your body's hunger and fullness cues, and eat until you feel satisfied, not overly full.

- Customize the meal plan and recipes to suit your preferences, dietary restrictions, and nutritional needs.

- Prioritize whole, nutrient-dense foods and minimize processed foods, refined sugars, and artificial ingredients.

- Consult with a healthcare professional before starting any new dietary regimen, especially if you have any underlying health conditions or concerns.

By following this 7-day detox meal plan and incorporating nourishing, wholesome foods into your diet, you can support your body's natural detoxification processes, boost energy levels, and promote overall health and well-being. Cheers to a rejuvenated and revitalized you!

CHAPTER SEVEN

Incorporating Detoxifying Practices into Your Routine

Detoxifying practices can play a vital role in supporting the body's natural cleansing processes, promoting overall health, and enhancing well-being. By incorporating these practices into your daily routine, you can help eliminate toxins, reduce inflammation, boost energy levels, and improve overall vitality. Here are several effective detoxifying practices that you can integrate into your routine:

1. Hydration

Staying hydrated is essential for supporting detoxification as it helps flush out toxins from the body, promote healthy digestion, and maintain optimal cellular function. Aim to drink plenty of water throughout the day, preferably filtered water to minimize exposure to contaminants. You can also incorporate hydrating beverages such as herbal teas, infused water, coconut water, and green juices to increase your fluid intake and support detoxification.

2. Healthy Eating

A balanced and nutrient-rich diet is crucial for supporting detoxification and promoting overall health. Focus on incorporating whole, plant-based foods such as fruits, vegetables, leafy greens, whole grains, legumes, nuts, and seeds into your meals. These foods are rich in antioxidants, vitamins, minerals, fiber, and phytonutrients that support liver function, aid digestion, and help eliminate toxins from the body. Minimize processed foods, refined sugars, artificial additives, and inflammatory foods that can burden the body's detoxification pathways and contribute to toxin buildup.

3. Regular Exercise

Regular physical activity is not only essential for maintaining a healthy weight and cardiovascular health but also for supporting detoxification. Exercise stimulates circulation, promotes sweating, and enhances lymphatic drainage, all of which help eliminate toxins from the body. Incorporate a variety of aerobic exercises, strength training, yoga, and flexibility exercises into your routine to promote overall fitness and detoxification. Aim for at least 30 minutes of moderate-intensity exercise most days of the week.

4. Deep Breathing

Practicing deep breathing exercises can help reduce stress, support relaxation, and enhance detoxification. Deep breathing stimulates the lymphatic system, increases oxygenation of tissues, and promotes the release of toxins through respiration. Incorporate deep breathing techniques such as diaphragmatic breathing, alternate nostril breathing, and belly breathing into your daily routine, especially during times of stress or tension.

5. Dry Brushing

Dry brushing is a technique that involves using a natural bristle brush to gently exfoliate the skin and stimulate the lymphatic system. Dry brushing helps remove dead skin cells, improve circulation, and promote lymphatic drainage, which can aid in detoxification. Before showering, use a dry brush to gently brush your skin in long, upward strokes, starting from your feet and moving towards your heart. Repeat this process for several minutes, then shower as usual.

6. Sauna Therapy

Sauna therapy is a popular detoxification practice that involves exposing the body to dry heat in a sauna or steam room. Sweating induced by sauna therapy helps eliminate toxins, heavy metals, and metabolic waste products through the skin. Regular sauna sessions can support detoxification, improve circulation, promote relaxation, and enhance overall well-being. Aim to incorporate sauna therapy into your routine once or twice a week, following safety guidelines and staying hydrated before, during, and after each session.

7. Herbal Support

Certain herbs and botanicals have detoxifying properties that can support liver function, aid digestion, and promote detoxification. Incorporate herbal teas, tinctures, or supplements containing detoxifying herbs such as dandelion root, milk thistle, burdock root, ginger, turmeric, and nettle into your routine to enhance detoxification and overall health. Consult with a healthcare professional or herbalist to determine the most appropriate herbs and dosages for your individual needs.

8. Mindfulness and Stress Management

Chronic stress can impair detoxification pathways and compromise overall health. Practicing mindfulness techniques such as meditation, deep breathing, yoga, tai chi, and progressive muscle relaxation can help reduce stress, support relaxation, and enhance detoxification. Schedule regular breaks throughout the day to practice mindfulness and stress management techniques, prioritize self-care activities, and cultivate a positive mindset to support your body's natural detoxification processes.

9. Adequate Sleep

Quality sleep is essential for supporting detoxification, cellular repair, and overall health. Aim to get seven to nine hours of restful sleep each night to allow your body to repair and regenerate. Create a relaxing bedtime routine, establish a consistent sleep schedule, optimize your sleep environment, and minimize exposure to electronic devices and stimulating activities before bedtime to promote deep, restorative sleep.

10. Limit Exposure to Toxins

Minimizing exposure to environmental toxins can help reduce the burden on your body's detoxification pathways and support overall health. Avoid or reduce exposure to common toxins found in pesticides, household cleaners, personal care products, plastics, and pollutants. Opt for natural and organic alternatives whenever possible, use air purifiers and water filters to reduce indoor pollution, and practice proper ventilation and ventilation to promote clean air quality in your home and workplace.

Incorporating these detoxifying practices into your daily routine can help support your body's natural cleansing processes, promote overall health, and enhance well-being. By making conscious choices to prioritize hydration, healthy eating, regular exercise, stress management, and toxin avoidance, you can optimize your body's ability to eliminate toxins and thrive in today's modern world.

CHAPTER EIGHT

Hydration and Supplements for Optimal Detox Results

Proper hydration and targeted supplementation play crucial roles in supporting the body's detoxification processes, promoting overall health, and maximizing the effectiveness of a detox program. By ensuring adequate hydration and incorporating key supplements, you can enhance detoxification, support organ function, and optimize cellular health. Here's a comprehensive guide to hydration and supplements for optimal detox results:

Hydration:

Hydration is fundamental to detoxification as it facilitates the elimination of toxins from the body, supports cellular function, and maintains overall hydration status. Adequate hydration is essential for optimal organ function, including the liver and kidneys, which are primary detoxification organs. Here are some tips to optimize hydration during a detox program:

1. **Water Intake:** Drink plenty of water throughout the day to support detoxification and maintain hydration. Aim for at least eight glasses of water daily, or more depending on your body size, activity level, and climate.

2. **Electrolyte Balance:** Electrolytes such as sodium, potassium, magnesium, and calcium are essential for maintaining fluid

balance, nerve function, and muscle contraction. Ensure adequate electrolyte intake by consuming electrolyte-rich foods such as fruits, vegetables, nuts, seeds, and electrolyte supplements as needed.

3. **Herbal Teas:** Incorporate hydrating herbal teas such as dandelion root tea, nettle tea, green tea, and peppermint tea into your daily routine. Herbal teas not only provide hydration but also offer additional health benefits, including liver support and antioxidant protection.

4. **Infused Water:** Enhance the flavor and nutritional value of water by infusing it with fresh fruits, herbs, and vegetables. Try adding slices of lemon, cucumber, mint, or berries to your water for a refreshing and hydrating beverage.

5. **Coconut Water:** Coconut water is a natural source of electrolytes, including potassium, magnesium, and sodium, making it an excellent hydrating beverage during a detox. Enjoy coconut water as a refreshing alternative to plain water to replenish electrolytes and support hydration.

6. **Hydration Tracking:** Monitor your hydration status by paying attention to signs of dehydration such as dry mouth, dark urine, fatigue, and headaches. Keep track of your water intake and aim to maintain a consistent level of hydration throughout the day.

Supplements for Optimal Detox Results:

In addition to hydration, targeted supplementation can enhance detoxification, support organ function, and address specific nutritional needs during a detox program. While it's important to obtain nutrients from whole foods whenever possible, certain supplements can complement a detox regimen and promote overall health. Here are some key supplements to consider for optimal detox results:

1. **Multivitamin and Mineral Complex:** A high-quality multivitamin and mineral supplement can provide essential nutrients needed for detoxification, including vitamins A, C, E, B vitamins, zinc, selenium, and magnesium. Choose a supplement that contains a comprehensive blend of vitamins and minerals to support overall health and fill nutritional gaps.

2. **Omega-3 Fatty Acids:** Omega-3 fatty acids, found in fish oil or algae supplements, are essential for supporting cellular health, reducing inflammation, and promoting detoxification. Incorporating omega-3 supplements can help balance omega-3 to omega-6 fatty acid ratios and support optimal brain function and cardiovascular health.

3. **Probiotics:** Probiotic supplements containing beneficial bacteria such as Lactobacillus and Bifidobacterium strains can support gut health, improve digestion, and enhance

detoxification. Probiotics help maintain a healthy balance of gut bacteria, which is essential for proper nutrient absorption, immune function, and toxin elimination.

4. **Liver Support Supplements:** Certain herbs and nutrients have been shown to support liver function and enhance detoxification pathways. Milk thistle, dandelion root, turmeric, N-acetylcysteine (NAC), and alpha-lipoic acid are examples of supplements that can support liver health, promote bile production, and facilitate toxin elimination.

5. **Antioxidants:** Antioxidant supplements such as vitamin C, vitamin E, selenium, glutathione, and alpha-lipoic acid can help neutralize free radicals, reduce oxidative stress, and protect cells from damage during detoxification. Incorporating antioxidant-rich foods and supplements can enhance detoxification and support overall health.

6. **Digestive Enzymes:** Digestive enzyme supplements can support optimal digestion and nutrient absorption, especially during periods of dietary change or increased fiber intake. Enzymes such as amylase, protease, lipase, and cellulase help break down carbohydrates, proteins, fats, and fiber, improving nutrient assimilation and reducing digestive discomfort.

7. **Detoxifying Herbs:** Certain herbs and botanicals have detoxifying properties that can support liver function, aid

digestion, and promote toxin elimination. Consider incorporating herbal supplements such as dandelion root, milk thistle, burdock root, ginger, turmeric, and cilantro into your detox regimen to enhance detoxification and support overall health.

8. **Adaptogens:** Adaptogenic herbs such as ashwagandha, rhodiola, holy basil, and astragalus can help reduce stress, support adrenal function, and enhance resilience to environmental stressors during a detox. Incorporating adaptogen supplements can support overall well-being and help mitigate the effects of stress on detoxification pathways.

Before starting any new supplementation regimen, it's essential to consult with a healthcare professional or qualified nutritionist to determine your individual nutrient needs, assess potential interactions with medications or existing health conditions, and ensure safe and effective use of supplements. Additionally, prioritize obtaining nutrients from whole foods whenever possible and focus on maintaining a balanced and nutrient-rich diet to support detoxification and overall health.

By prioritizing hydration and incorporating targeted supplements into your detox regimen, you can support the body's natural detoxification processes, promote optimal organ function, and enhance overall health and vitality. Combine these strategies with healthy eating, regular exercise, stress management techniques, and adequate sleep to optimize your detox results and cultivate a vibrant and resilient body.

CHAPTER NINE

Addressing Detox Symptoms and Challenges

Embarking on a detoxification journey can bring about various symptoms and challenges as your body adjusts to dietary and lifestyle changes, eliminates toxins, and undergoes physiological shifts. It's essential to understand common detox symptoms and challenges and implement strategies to address them effectively. By proactively managing detox symptoms and challenges, you can optimize your detox experience and support overall well-being. Here's a comprehensive guide to addressing detox symptoms and challenges:

1. Common Detox Symptoms:

a. Headaches: Headaches are a common detox symptom and may occur due to caffeine withdrawal, dehydration, changes in blood sugar levels, or the release of toxins from fat cells. Stay hydrated, gradually reduce caffeine intake, practice stress management techniques, and consider using natural remedies such as peppermint oil or ginger tea to alleviate headaches.

b. Fatigue: Fatigue is often experienced during detox as the body redirects energy towards detoxification processes. Ensure adequate rest and sleep, prioritize relaxation and stress management techniques, consume nutrient-dense foods to support energy levels, and consider incorporating adaptogenic herbs or supplements to support adrenal function and reduce fatigue.

c. Digestive Issues: Digestive issues such as bloating, gas, constipation, or diarrhea may arise as your body adjusts to dietary changes and increased fiber intake. Eat smaller, frequent meals, chew food thoroughly, consume plenty of fiber-rich foods, stay hydrated, incorporate digestive enzymes or probiotics to support gut health, and avoid triggering foods that exacerbate digestive discomfort.

d. Skin Breakouts: Skin breakouts or acne may occur as the body eliminates toxins through the skin. Practice proper skincare, cleanse your skin regularly, avoid harsh chemicals or skincare products, stay hydrated, consume a nutrient-rich diet, and consider incorporating detoxifying herbs or supplements such as milk thistle or dandelion root to support liver function and promote clear skin.

e. Mood Swings: Mood swings, irritability, or emotional fluctuations may occur as the body undergoes detoxification and hormonal changes. Practice stress management techniques such as deep breathing, meditation, yoga, or tai chi, prioritize self-care activities, engage in gentle exercise, ensure adequate sleep, and seek support from friends, family, or a healthcare professional if needed.

2. Challenges During Detox:

a. Cravings: Cravings for unhealthy foods, sugar, caffeine, or processed snacks may arise during detox as the body adjusts to dietary changes and withdrawals from addictive substances. Practice mindful eating, identify triggers for cravings, substitute healthier alternatives, stay hydrated, consume nutrient-dense foods to satisfy hunger, and distract yourself with enjoyable activities or hobbies.

b. Social Pressure: Social situations or peer pressure may present challenges during detox, especially when dining out, attending social gatherings, or interacting with friends and family who may not understand or support your detox goals. Communicate your intentions and boundaries clearly, plan ahead by bringing your own nutritious snacks or meals, focus on socializing rather than food, and seek support from like-minded individuals or online communities.

c. Detox Plateaus: Detox plateaus occur when progress stalls, and you no longer experience significant improvements in energy, digestion, or other health markers despite following a detox program diligently. Reassess your detox protocol, incorporate additional detoxifying practices or supplements, prioritize stress management and relaxation techniques, ensure adequate sleep and hydration, and consider consulting with a healthcare professional or qualified nutritionist for personalized guidance.

d. Detox Herxheimer Reaction: A Herxheimer reaction, also known as a "healing crisis," may occur when the body experiences a temporary worsening of symptoms before improvement occurs. This reaction happens as toxins are released and eliminated from the body, leading to flu-like symptoms such as fatigue, muscle aches, headaches, or nausea. Support your body's detoxification processes with adequate hydration, rest, nutrient-dense foods, and gentle exercise, and consider incorporating supportive supplements or herbs to alleviate symptoms.

e. Emotional Release: Detoxification can sometimes trigger emotional releases or heightened sensitivity as stored emotions and psychological toxins are released along with physical toxins. Practice self-awareness, journaling, meditation, or mindfulness techniques to process emotions, seek support from a therapist or counselor if needed, prioritize self-care activities that promote relaxation and emotional well-being, and allow yourself to experience and express emotions in a healthy and constructive manner.

3. Strategies to Address Detox Symptoms and Challenges:

- **Gradual Transition:** Gradually transition into and out of a detox program to minimize shock to the body and reduce the severity of detox symptoms. Start by gradually reducing caffeine, sugar, processed foods, and other potential triggers before beginning the detox, and gradually reintroduce foods post-detox to identify any sensitivities or intolerances.

- **Listen to Your Body:** Pay attention to your body's signals and adjust your detox protocol accordingly. If certain foods or practices exacerbate symptoms or discomfort, modify your approach or seek alternative strategies that better suit your individual needs and preferences.

- **Supportive Therapies:** Incorporate supportive therapies such as massage, acupuncture, dry brushing, hydrotherapy, or sauna sessions to enhance detoxification, promote relaxation, and alleviate detox symptoms. These therapies can support circulation, lymphatic drainage, and toxin elimination, facilitating a smoother detox experience.

- **Professional Guidance:** Seek guidance from a qualified healthcare professional, nutritionist, or functional medicine practitioner who can provide personalized recommendations, monitor your progress, and address any concerns or challenges that arise during the detoxification process.

- **Mind-Body Practices:** Engage in mind-body practices such as yoga, meditation, deep breathing, progressive muscle relaxation, or guided imagery to reduce stress, promote relaxation, and enhance overall well-being during detox. These practices can help modulate the body's stress response, support emotional balance, and facilitate detoxification.

- **Celebrate Progress:** Celebrate small victories and milestones along your detox journey, whether it's improved energy levels, clearer skin, better digestion, or enhanced mood. Acknowledge your efforts and progress, and recognize that each step forward, no matter how small, contributes to your overall health and well-being.

Conclusion:

Addressing detox symptoms and challenges requires a multifaceted approach that prioritizes self-care, flexibility, and resilience. By understanding common detox symptoms, proactively managing challenges, and implementing supportive strategies, you can optimize your detox experience, support your body's natural detoxification processes, and promote overall health and vitality. Remember to listen to your body, honor your individual needs, and seek support when needed to navigate

Transitioning Out of the Detox: Post-Detox Guidelines and Long-Term Health Strategies

Completing a detox program is a significant accomplishment, but transitioning out of the detox phase is equally important to maintain the benefits achieved and support long-term health and well-being. Post-detox guidelines and long-term health strategies play a crucial role in sustaining the positive changes initiated during the detox period, promoting continued detoxification, and cultivating a lifestyle that supports optimal health. Here's a comprehensive guide to transitioning out of the detox phase and implementing long-term health strategies:

1. Gradual Reintroduction of Foods:

After completing a detox program, reintroduce foods gradually to identify any potential sensitivities, allergies, or intolerances. Start with easily digestible foods such as steamed vegetables, lean proteins, whole grains, and fruits, and gradually reintroduce other foods while paying attention to how your body responds. Keep a food journal to track your symptoms and make informed dietary choices based on your individual tolerance and preferences.

2. Balanced and Nutrient-Rich Diet:

Transition to a balanced and nutrient-rich diet that prioritizes whole, unprocessed foods, and incorporates a variety of fruits, vegetables, leafy greens, whole grains, legumes, nuts, seeds, lean proteins, and healthy fats. Focus on incorporating a rainbow of colorful fruits and vegetables to maximize nutrient intake and antioxidant protection, and prioritize organic and locally sourced foods whenever possible to minimize exposure to pesticides and contaminants.

3. Hydration and Detox Support:

Continue to prioritize hydration and support detoxification by maintaining adequate water intake, consuming hydrating beverages such as herbal teas and coconut water, and incorporating detoxifying foods and supplements into your diet. Consider incorporating foods and herbs known for their detoxifying properties, such as cruciferous vegetables, leafy greens, garlic, ginger, turmeric, and cilantro, to support liver function and promote toxin elimination.

4. Regular Physical Activity:

Maintain a regular exercise routine that includes a combination of cardiovascular exercise, strength training, flexibility exercises, and mind-body practices such as yoga or tai chi. Exercise promotes circulation, lymphatic drainage, and sweating, all of which support detoxification and overall health. Aim for at least 150 minutes of moderate-intensity exercise per week, and prioritize activities that you enjoy and can sustain long term.

5. Stress Management and Self-Care:

Prioritize stress management techniques and self-care practices to support overall well-being and reduce the impact of stress on your health. Incorporate relaxation techniques such as meditation, deep breathing, progressive muscle relaxation, or guided imagery into your daily routine, and prioritize activities that promote relaxation and joy, such as spending time in nature, practicing hobbies, or connecting with loved ones.

6. Adequate Sleep and Rest:

Ensure adequate sleep and rest to support cellular repair, hormone balance, and overall health. Aim for seven to nine hours of restful sleep per night, establish a consistent sleep schedule, create a relaxing bedtime routine, and optimize your sleep environment by minimizing noise, light, and electronic devices. Prioritize quality sleep as an essential component of long-term health and well-being.

7. Mindful Eating and Intuitive Eating:

Practice mindful eating and intuitive eating principles to cultivate a positive relationship with food, listen to your body's hunger and fullness cues, and make nourishing food choices that honor your physical and emotional needs. Slow down during meals, savor the flavors and textures of your food, and tune into your body's signals to guide your eating patterns. Focus on nourishing your body with nutrient-dense foods that support your health and vitality.

8. Continued Detoxification Practices:

Incorporate ongoing detoxification practices into your daily routine to support the body's natural cleansing processes and promote overall health. Consider incorporating practices such as dry brushing, sauna therapy, hydrotherapy, or lymphatic massage to support detoxification and promote lymphatic drainage. Additionally, continue to prioritize hydration, consume antioxidant-rich foods, and support liver function with herbs and supplements to maintain optimal detoxification.

9. Regular Health Assessments:

Schedule regular health assessments with your healthcare provider to monitor your progress, assess key health markers, and address any emerging health concerns. Stay proactive about your health by scheduling routine check-ups, screenings, and laboratory tests as recommended based on your age, gender, family history, and lifestyle factors. Discuss your detox experience and long-term health goals with your healthcare provider to develop a personalized health plan that aligns with your needs and priorities.

10. Consistency and Sustainability:

Focus on consistency and sustainability in your health habits and lifestyle choices to support long-term health and well-being. Embrace gradual changes and small, sustainable habits that you can maintain over time, rather than quick fixes or extreme approaches that are difficult to sustain. Cultivate a balanced approach to health that prioritizes self-care, moderation, flexibility, and enjoyment, and be kind to yourself as you navigate your health journey.

Conclusion:

Transitioning out of the detox phase is a critical step in maintaining the benefits achieved and supporting long-term health and vitality. By implementing post-detox guidelines and long-term health strategies, you can continue to support detoxification, promote overall health, and cultivate a lifestyle that aligns with your health goals and values. Prioritize balanced nutrition, regular physical activity, stress management, adequate sleep, and ongoing detoxification practices to optimize your health and well-being for the long term. Remember that your health journey is unique to you, and it's essential to listen to your body, honor your individual needs, and seek support when needed as you navigate your path to wellness.

BONUS

SOME HERBAL APPROACHES TO KNOW

Manjakani:

Definition: Manjakani, also known as Quercus infectoria or oak gall, is a natural substance derived from the oak tree. It has been used for centuries in traditional medicine for its potential health benefits, particularly for women's health and vaginal tightening.

Ingredients: Manjakani contains various bioactive compounds, including tannins, flavonoids, and gallic acid. These compounds are believed to contribute to the herb's medicinal properties, including its potential as an astringent and antiseptic agent.

How to Prepare: Manjakani is typically available in powder, capsule, or liquid extract form. It can be taken orally or used topically depending on the intended use. For vaginal tightening, manjakani may be applied topically as a gel or inserted into the vagina in capsule form.

Dosage: The appropriate dosage of manjakani can vary depending on factors such as age, health status, and the specific preparation being used. It's important to follow the recommended dosage on the product label or consult with a qualified herbalist or healthcare professional for personalized guidance.

How to Use: Manjakani can be taken orally or used topically depending on the intended use. It's important to use manjakani products as directed and to discontinue use if any adverse effects occur.

Side Effects: Manjakani is generally considered safe for most people when used in moderate amounts. However, some individuals may experience allergic reactions or skin irritation when used topically. It's important to use manjakani under the guidance of a healthcare professional and to discontinue use if any adverse effects occur.

Red Clover:

Definition: Red clover, scientifically known as Trifolium pratense, is a flowering plant belonging to the legume family. It's native to Europe, Western Asia, and Northwest Africa but has been naturalized in many other regions. Red clover has been used in traditional medicine for various purposes, including its potential to support women's health and menopausal symptoms.

Ingredients: Red clover contains several bioactive compounds, including isoflavones (such as genistein and daidzein), flavonoids, and phytoestrogens. These compounds are believed to contribute to the herb's medicinal properties, including its potential as a hormone-balancing agent and its ability to support cardiovascular health.

How to Prepare: Red clover is typically prepared and consumed as an herbal tea or tincture. To make tea, dried red clover flowers are steeped in hot water for several minutes before being strained and consumed. Tinctures are prepared by steeping the flowers in alcohol or vinegar to extract their active compounds.

Dosage: The appropriate dosage of red clover can vary depending on factors such as age, health status, and the specific preparation being used. It's important to follow the recommended dosage on the product label or consult with a qualified herbalist or healthcare professional for personalized guidance.

How to Use: Red clover tea or tincture is typically taken orally. It's important to use red clover products as directed and to discontinue use if any adverse effects occur.

Side Effects: Red clover is generally considered safe for most people when used in moderate amounts. However, some individuals may experience allergic reactions or digestive upset. It may also interact with certain medications or have adverse effects in individuals with certain health conditions. It's important to use red clover under the guidance of a healthcare professional and to discontinue use if any adverse effects occur.

Red Raspberry:

Definition: Red raspberry, scientifically known as Rubus idaeus, is a species of raspberry native to Europe and northern Asia. It's widely cultivated for its delicious berries and has been used in traditional medicine for various purposes, including its potential to support women's health during pregnancy and childbirth.

Ingredients: Red raspberry contains several bioactive compounds, including flavonoids, ellagic acid, anthocyanins, and vitamin C. These compounds are believed to contribute to the herb's medicinal properties, including its potential as an antioxidant, anti-inflammatory, and uterine tonic.

How to Prepare: Red raspberry leaf is typically prepared and consumed as an herbal tea or infusion. To make tea, dried red raspberry leaves are steeped in hot water for several minutes before being strained and consumed.

Dosage: The appropriate dosage of red raspberry leaf can vary depending on factors such as age, health status, and the specific preparation being used. It's important to follow the recommended dosage on the product label or consult with a qualified herbalist or healthcare professional for personalized guidance.

How to Use: Red raspberry leaf tea is typically taken orally. It's often recommended for pregnant individuals in the later stages of pregnancy to support uterine health and prepare for childbirth. It's important to use red raspberry leaf products as directed and to discontinue use if any adverse effects occur.

Side Effects: Red raspberry leaf is generally considered safe for most people when used in moderate amounts. However, some individuals may experience allergic reactions or digestive upset. Pregnant individuals should consult with a healthcare professional before using red raspberry leaf, especially if they have any underlying health conditions or are taking medications. It's important to use red raspberry leaf under the guidance of a healthcare professional and to discontinue use if any adverse effects occur.

Rhubarb:

Definition: Rhubarb, scientifically known as Rheum rhabarbarum, is a perennial plant cultivated for its edible stalks. While primarily used in culinary applications, rhubarb has also been utilized in traditional medicine for its potential health benefits, particularly for digestive health.

Ingredients: Rhubarb stalks contain various bioactive compounds, including anthraquinones (such as emodin and rhein), fiber, vitamins (such as vitamin K), and minerals (including calcium and potassium). These compounds are believed to contribute to the herb's medicinal properties, including its potential as a laxative and digestive aid.

How to Prepare: Rhubarb stalks are typically cooked before consumption, as the raw stalks are very tart and can be unpleasant to eat. They are often used in pies, crisps, jams, sauces, and other desserts, as well as in savory dishes. Rhubarb can also be used to make compotes, jams, and preserves.

Dosage: There is no specific dosage for rhubarb in culinary applications, as it is used as a food rather than a medicinal herb. However, when used for its potential laxative effects, it's important to consume rhubarb in moderation to avoid gastrointestinal upset.

How to Use: Rhubarb stalks can be chopped and cooked in various dishes, including pies, sauces, and jams. It's important to remove and discard the leaves, as they contain toxic compounds. When using rhubarb for its potential laxative effects, it's typically consumed as part of a cooked dish or in the form of a rhubarb-based herbal remedy.

Side Effects: Rhubarb stalks are generally safe for most people when consumed in moderate amounts as part of a balanced diet. However, excessive intake may lead to digestive upset or adverse effects due to the presence of oxalic acid, which can bind to calcium and form kidney stones in susceptible individuals. It's important to use rhubarb in moderation and to consult with a healthcare professional if you have any concerns or underlying health conditions.

Sarsaparilla:

Definition: Sarsaparilla refers to several species of plants belonging to the Smilax genus, including Smilax regelii and Smilax officinalis. It has been used historically in traditional medicine for its potential health benefits, particularly for its purported detoxifying and anti-inflammatory properties.

Ingredients: Sarsaparilla contains various bioactive compounds, including saponins (such as sarsaponin and smilagenin), flavonoids, phenolic acids, and sterols. These compounds are believed to contribute to the herb's medicinal properties, including its potential as a diuretic, blood purifier, and anti-inflammatory agent.

How to Prepare: Sarsaparilla root is typically prepared and consumed as an herbal tea, decoction, or tincture. To make tea, dried sarsaparilla root is steeped in hot water for several minutes before being strained and consumed. Decoctions involve boiling the root in water to extract its active compounds, while tinctures are prepared by steeping the root in alcohol or vinegar.

Dosage: The appropriate dosage of sarsaparilla can vary depending on factors such as age, health status, and the specific preparation being used. It's important to follow the recommended dosage on the product label or consult with a qualified herbalist or healthcare professional for personalized guidance.

How to Use: Sarsaparilla tea or tincture is typically taken orally. It's important to use sarsaparilla products as directed and to discontinue use if any adverse effects occur.

Side Effects: Sarsaparilla is generally considered safe for most people when used in moderate amounts. However, some individuals may experience allergic reactions or digestive upset. It may also interact with certain medications or have adverse effects in individuals with certain health conditions. It's important to use sarsaparilla under the guidance of a healthcare professional and to discontinue use if any adverse effects occur.

Tila:

Definition: Tila, also known as linden flower or lime blossom, refers to the flowers of the Tilia genus, primarily Tilia europaea and Tilia cordata. These trees are native to Europe, but they are also cultivated in other regions for their fragrant and medicinal flowers.

Ingredients: Tila flowers contain various bioactive compounds, including flavonoids, phenolic acids, and volatile oils. These compounds are believed to contribute to the herb's medicinal properties, including its potential as a mild sedative, anxiolytic, and anti-inflammatory agent.

How to Prepare: Tila flowers are typically prepared and consumed as an herbal tea or infusion. To make tea, dried tila flowers are steeped in hot water for several minutes before being strained and consumed.

Dosage: The appropriate dosage of tila can vary depending on factors such as age, health status, and the specific preparation being used. It's important to follow the recommended dosage on the product label or consult with a qualified herbalist or healthcare professional for personalized guidance.

How to Use: Tila tea is typically taken orally. It's often consumed in the evening as a calming bedtime beverage or during times of stress or anxiety. It's important to use tila products as directed and to discontinue use if any adverse effects occur.

Side Effects: Tila is generally considered safe for most people when used in moderate amounts. However, some individuals may experience allergic reactions or digestive upset. It may also interact with certain medications or have adverse effects in individuals with certain health conditions. It's important to use tila under the guidance of a healthcare professional and to discontinue use if any adverse effects occur.

Valerian:

Definition: Valerian, scientifically known as Valeriana officinalis, is a perennial flowering plant native to Europe and Asia. It has been used for centuries in traditional medicine for its potential calming and sedative effects.

Ingredients: Valerian root contains several bioactive compounds, including valerenic acid, valepotriates, and volatile oils. These compounds are believed to contribute to the herb's medicinal properties, including its potential as a sedative, anxiolytic, and sleep aid.

How to Prepare: Valerian root is typically prepared and consumed as an herbal tea, tincture, or capsule. To make tea, dried valerian root is steeped in hot water for several minutes before being strained and consumed. Tinctures are prepared by steeping the root in alcohol or vinegar to extract its active compounds.

Dosage: The appropriate dosage of valerian can vary depending on factors such as age, health status, and the specific preparation being used. It's important to follow the recommended dosage on the product label or consult with a qualified herbalist or healthcare professional for personalized guidance.

How to Use: Valerian tea, tincture, or capsules are typically taken orally. It's often consumed in the evening as a sleep aid or during times of stress or anxiety. It's important to use valerian products as directed and to discontinue use if any adverse effects occur.

Side Effects: Valerian is generally considered safe for most people when used in moderate amounts. However, some individuals may experience mild side effects such as drowsiness, headache, or gastrointestinal upset. It may also interact with certain medications or have adverse effects in individuals with certain health conditions. It's important to use valerian under the guidance of a healthcare professional and to discontinue use if any adverse effects occur.

Wild Cherry Bark:

Definition: Wild cherry bark, scientifically known as Prunus serotina, is the bark obtained from the black cherry tree native to North America. It has been used traditionally in Native American and folk medicine for its potential health benefits, particularly for respiratory and digestive issues.

Ingredients: Wild cherry bark contains various bioactive compounds, including cyanogenic glycosides (such as prunasin and amygdalin), flavonoids, and phenolic acids. These compounds are believed to contribute to the herb's medicinal properties, including its potential as an expectorant, cough suppressant, and mild sedative.

How to Prepare: Wild cherry bark is typically prepared and consumed as an herbal tea, decoction, or syrup. To make tea, dried wild cherry bark is steeped in hot water for several minutes before being strained and consumed. Decoctions involve boiling the bark in water to extract its active compounds, while syrups are made by simmering the bark with sugar or honey to create a thick, sweet liquid.

Dosage: The appropriate dosage of wild cherry bark can vary depending on factors such as age, health status, and the specific preparation being used. It's important to follow the recommended dosage on the product label or consult with a qualified herbalist or healthcare professional for personalized guidance.

How to Use: Wild cherry bark tea, decoction, or syrup is typically taken orally. It's often consumed to soothe coughs, sore throats, and other respiratory symptoms. It's important to use wild cherry bark products as directed and to discontinue use if any adverse effects occur.

Side Effects: Wild cherry bark is generally considered safe for most people when used in moderate amounts. However, it contains cyanogenic glycosides, which can release cyanide in the body when metabolized. While the risk of cyanide poisoning from consuming wild cherry bark is low when used appropriately, excessive intake or prolonged use may lead to adverse effects. It's important to use wild cherry bark under the guidance of a healthcare professional and to discontinue use if any adverse effects occur.

Black Cohosh:

Definition: Black cohosh, scientifically known as Actaea racemosa (formerly Cimicifuga racemosa), is a perennial herb native to North America. It has a long history of use in traditional Native American medicine and later in folk medicine for its potential health benefits, particularly for women's health.

Ingredients: Black cohosh root contains various bioactive compounds, including triterpene glycosides (such as actein and cimicifugoside), phenolic acids, and flavonoids. These compounds are believed to contribute to the herb's medicinal properties, including its potential as a hormone-balancing agent and its ability to relieve menopausal symptoms.

How to Prepare: Black cohosh is typically consumed as a powdered root, herbal tea, tincture, or in supplement form (such as capsules or tablets). To make tea, dried black cohosh root is steeped in hot water for several minutes before being strained and consumed.

Dosage: The appropriate dosage of black cohosh can vary depending on factors such as age, health status, and the specific preparation being used. It's important to follow the recommended dosage on the product label or consult with a qualified herbalist or healthcare professional for personalized guidance.

How to Use: Black cohosh powder, tea, tincture, or supplements are typically taken orally. It's often used by women to support hormonal balance, relieve menopausal symptoms such as hot flashes and night sweats, and promote overall well-being.

Side Effects: Black cohosh is generally considered safe for most people when used in moderate amounts. However, some individuals may experience mild side effects such as gastrointestinal upset or allergic reactions. It may also interact with certain medications or have adverse effects in individuals with certain health conditions, such as liver disease or hormone-sensitive conditions. Pregnant or breastfeeding individuals should consult with a healthcare professional before using black cohosh supplements. It's important to use black cohosh under the guidance of a healthcare professional and to discontinue use if any adverse effects occur.

THE END